Grieving for Your Hearing Loss

The Rocky Road from Denial to Acceptance

Third Edition

Neil G. Bauman, Ph.D.

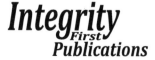

Lynden, WA   http://IntegrityFirstPublications.com

Grieving for Your Hearing Loss
The Rocky Road from Denial to Acceptance

Third Edition

Another **Integrity First** book in the series:

Everything You Wanted to Know About Your Hearing Loss But Were Afraid to Ask
(Because You Knew You Wouldn't Hear the Answers Anyway!)

Copyright   1997, 2000, 2011 by Neil G. Bauman

ISBN 978-1-935939-10-8

All rights reserved. No part of this publication may be reproduced or transmitted in any form or by any means, electronic or mechanical, including photocopying, recording or any other information storage and retrieval system without permission in writing from the publisher, except by a reviewer who may quote brief passages in a review.

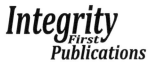

Publications

1013 Ridgeway Drive,
Lynden, WA 98264-1057
Phone: (360) 778-1266
FAX: (360) 389-5226
Email: info@IntegrityFirstPublications.com
Website: http://IntegrityFirstPublications.com

Printed in the United States of America

Warning—Disclaimer

This book is for your education and reference. It is neither a medical manual nor a guide to self-treatment for medical problems. Do not construe this book as giving personal medical advice or instruction. The author is not a medical doctor and neither prescribes treatment nor treats medical problems and does not intend that you attempt to do so either. If you suspect that you have a medical problem related to your ears, seek competent professional medical help. Use the information in this book to help you make informed decisions, not as a substitute for any treatment that your doctor may have prescribed for you.

The information and opinions expressed in this book are the result of careful research. They are believed to be accurate and sound, based on the best judgment available to the author. If you fail to consult appropriate health professionals, you assume the risk of any injuries. Neither Integrity First Publications, the Center for Hearing Loss Help, nor the author assumes any responsibility for damages or losses incurred as a result of using the information in this book, nor for any errors or omissions. It is the responsibility of each reader to exercise good judgment in using any information contained in this book.

Contents

About the Author 7

Preface 9

1. **Grieving for Your Hearing Loss** 11
   What Is Grief? 12
   The Work of Grieving 14
   Ignoring Grief Also Brings Results—
      Negative Results 18
   The Stages of Grief 20

2. **Denial** 23

3. **Anger** 31

4. **Bargaining** 35

5. **Depression** 37

6. **Acceptance** 43

7. **Grieving and Your Family** **47**
    The Rest of Your Family Needs to
        Grieve Too 47
    Where Does Getting Hearing Aids Fit
        into the Grieving Process? 49

Literature Cited..**53**

Good Books on Hearing Loss...............................**57**

About the Author

Neil G. Bauman, Ph.D., (Dr. Neil), is the C.E.O. of the Center for Hearing Loss Help. He is a hearing loss coping skills specialist, researcher, author and speaker on issues pertaining to hearing loss. No stranger to hearing loss himself, he has lived with a life-long, severe, hereditary hearing loss.

Dr. Neil did not let his hearing loss stop him from achieving what he wanted to do. He earned several degrees in fields ranging from forestry to ancient astronomy (Ph. D.) and theology (Th. D.) in addition to his extensive studies in fields related to hearing loss.

His mission is helping hard of hearing people understand and successfully cope with their hearing losses and other ear conditions. To this end, he provides education, support and counsel to hard of hearing people through personal contact, as well as through his books, articles, presentations and seminars.

Dr. Neil is the author of eleven books and more than 1,000 articles on hearing-loss related topics.

(See the back of this book for a list of his books.) In addition, he is a dynamic speaker. His presentations are in demand throughout the USA and Canada.

He is a member of the Hearing Loss Association of America and the Canadian Hard of Hearing Association.

You can reach him at:

Neil Bauman, Ph.D.
Center for Hearing Loss Help
1013 Ridgeway Drive
Lynden, WA 98264-1057
Phone: (360) 778-1266
FAX: (260) 389-5226
Email: neil@hearinglosshelp.com
Web site: http://hearinglosshelp.com

Preface

When we finally (or perhaps suddenly) realize that we are losing or have lost much of our hearing, our emotional systems receive a terrific shock. Later, our emotional systems receive another shock when we realize that nobody can do anything to restore our hearing—that it's a life sentence. We will never hear better than we do now. We need to find a way to cope with this emotional turmoil. The right way to do this is by grieving for our hearing loss.

If this is your situation, this book will help you.

Neil Bauman, Ph.D.
Lynden, WA

Chapter 1

Grieving for Your Hearing Loss

When we lose some, much, or all of our hearing, especially if it is reasonably sudden, we are thrown into emotional turmoil whether we admit it or not.

We cope with our losses one way or another. Some of us do the right things, but unfortunately, many of us, at least initially, cope the wrong way—like Robin did. Here is her story.

Robin was a normal-hearing, 21-year-old young woman when she went to a sleep-over at a friend's house. Due to a tragic set of circumstances, she awoke the next morning totally deaf. She relates,

> "I walked out of my friend's house to get a ride home—they lived on a highway—and I saw a tractor-trailer go whizzing by, the trees, leaves and grass bending and swaying as the truck raced past me, but there was no sound. The lack of sound just did not compute to my brain. I was numb."

The tragedy of losing her hearing overnight turned Robin into a zombie as she struggled to deal with her loss.

What did she do? She explained,

"I shut myself up in my bedroom for 20 months!"

Why? She continued,

"I didn't know how to deal with this hearing loss. I didn't know anyone else who was hard of hearing. Furthermore, I refused to consider hearing aids."

No matter how you lose your hearing, once you become aware of your hearing loss, what you do next largely determines whether you will live a happy, fulfilled life as a hard of hearing person, or whether you have just set yourself up for all sorts of physical, emotional and psychological problems in the future like Robin did.

You don't have to be like Robin. You **can** successfully live with your hearing loss. But first you need to grieve—to work though the grieving process.

What Is Grief?

Grief is intense emotional suffering caused by a significant loss in our lives. It is a process we work through, not a state of being. Grief is a natural, necessary, healthy, human reaction. We value our hearing. Therefore, we quite naturally grieve its loss. Our grief shows that we recognize we have a hearing loss and that we are powerless to restore it.

No one denies that grief is painful. When we squarely face our hearing loss, the waves of emotions and feelings we call grief flow over us. Like waves of the sea, the grief process follows a natural course that builds and then recedes. This grieving process can't be rushed or turned back. As each wave of grief

Chapter 1: Grieving for Your Hearing Loss

rises and crests, we need to recognize our loss and experience the pain it brings. As each wave of grief subsides and recedes, we begin to adjust to those changes our hearing loss brings. Our emotions begin to heal. We begin to look to the future once more.

These waves of grief with their intense emotional, physical and mental under currents, will wash over us for some time. They will disturb our once normal lives. Our feelings may be so overwhelming that we may try to avoid them. We need to understand that the fear, sadness, crying, thinking about our loss, and other expressions of grief aren't us "breaking down". Not at all. We're "breaking through!"

Crying is a natural part of the grieving process. When we do not express our grief, we literally make ourselves sick.[1] So, if we resist these waves of grief like we may want to, or if we deny or minimize our pain, we only postpone the day we must ultimately face our grief.

Our grief normally waxes and wanes during the day. We may be joking with friends but half an hour later be distraught with waves of grief.[2] We must allow each wave to flow over us.

Normal physical reactions to grief can include difficulty sleeping or needing more sleep than usual, loss of appetite, tightness in our chest or throat, weakness, lack of energy and shortness of breath. Mentally we may feel fearful, preoccupied about our hearing loss, anxious, confused, forgetful and unable to concentrate.

Understanding the grieving process helps us face the reality of our losses. It helps us deal with our feelings of fear, loneliness, despair and helplessness. It helps us recover and grow through these experiences. As we learn to accept our grief we become stronger people. In time the pain goes away. We become capable of living happy, full lives once again.[3]

The Work of Grieving

Grief is the process of working through the tasks of grieving. Although these tasks are the same for all of us, each of us experiences grief differently because we are all unique. Here are the four tasks of grieving:

1. We must accept the reality of our losses.
2. We must experience the pain of grief.
3. We must accept and readjust to our new level of hearing.
4. We must redirect our emotional energy to achieving new goals in our lives.[4]

Part of the task of grieving is to set up new patterns of behavior. Before we can do that, we must give up those old ways that no longer work. This means discarding old patterns of communicating that now no longer work for us. In their place we must learn new ones that are appropriate for our hearing loss. This frees us from the past. It can be a long and painful process.[5] We are now ready to work towards finding fulfillment in the future.

The time each of us requires to work through our grief varies greatly. As long as we are making progress, this is not important. If we get "stuck" somewhere in the process, we should seek competent help. Note that time by itself will not heal our emotions. It is what we do with our time that makes the difference!

Chapter 1: Grieving for Your Hearing Loss

We never completely work through our hearing loss in the sense that we leave it behind. This is because each of us, as hard of hearing people, have an ongoing disability. As a result, our grief has no end point. We must daily handle the effects of our hearing loss.

While we normally grieve more at the beginning of our loss, our sorrow will last as long as we live. Each new change in our hearing loss may trigger a renewed grief cycle. Then, too, waves of grief can wash over us whenever something reminds us of our loss.[6] Although these waves of grief may continue for months or years, the waves usually become smaller and less frequent with time. How disruptive each wave will be depends on the strength of our support groups and how much our hearing changes.[7]

We do not like to grieve in public. When we grieve we want **safety**.

1. We need a **safe place** to grieve. Normally we want to withdraw to our own homes to grieve.

2. We need **safe people** around us while we are grieving. We need emotional support, especially with those who have gone through similar experiences.

3. We need **safe situations**. We need worthwhile activities where we can fully participate with people who also understand our sense of loss and grief.[8]

Here are some things we can do to help ourselves through our grief.

1. We need to express our feelings aloud. We need to openly admit our anxieties and fears. If we

hold painful feelings inside, they will create more problems for us later.

2. We need to accept help from those who offer it. The understanding and support of others can make our difficult moments easier. If we need help, we must ask for it. Often our relatives and friends want to help us, but often don't know quite what to do unless we tell them. We must be ready to seek professional help if we need it.

3. We need to be patient and kind to ourselves. Some days will be more difficult than others. We must continue to believe that we will recover.

4. We need to get plenty of rest each day. That way we will have more energy to handle life's problems and to get involved once again in activities we enjoy. Taking pride in our physical appearance lifts our spirits as well.

5. We need to keep ourselves healthy by eating balanced meals and exercising regularly. We should avoid alcohol, tranquilizers and other potentially harmful substances.[9]

> **Dr. Hawking's Formula for Success**
>
> Dr. Stephen Hawking, the famous astrophysicist who became completely paralyzed once said, "If you're disabled, you should pour your energies into those areas where you are not handicapped. You should concentrate on what you can do well, and not mourn over what you cannot do.
>
> It is very important not to give in to self-pity. If you're disabled and you feel sorry for yourself, then no one is going to have much to do with you. A physically handicapped person certainly can't afford to be psychologically handicapped as well."[10]

6. We need to begin doing productive things again. This can have a tremendous effect on how we feel about ourselves and the future. As a starter, we can set goals for ourselves and then work to reach them. We should start with simple, easy-to-accomplish, short-term goals. After we have developed successes with the short-term goals, we are then ready to develop long-range plans. We need to write down any goals we have for the future—for example, getting a new job, continuing our education or trying a new hobby.

> **Sam's Secret for Success**
>
> If we want to achieve the best that is possible for us, we need to participate in activities that use our strengths. We must focus on the things we are good at. We will have to exercise our strengths daily. This means practice, practice, practice. It is generally unproductive trying to bolster our weaknesses. Therefore, we should ignore our weaknesses unless they hinder us. By following this procedure, we will succeed.[11]

7. We need to check our progress periodically. We need to persevere. This means never, never give up.

8. We need to try new activities. Our hearing loss has changed our lives and given us the need for new direction. We might want to join a different club or organization that better fits in with our hearing loss. We need to be with people who have similar interests. Consider taking a course in a subject or skill you've always wanted to explore. Another rewarding area is to do some volunteer

work. By helping others, we may find that we are also helping ourselves as well. Perhaps it is time we changed our jobs to one better suited to our changed hearing.

9. Join a support group for people with hearing losses. Just being with others who also have hearing losses will help us. If there is no support group nearby, why not begin one? The purpose of such a group is not so you can wallow in self-pity with others in the same situation as yourself. Rather, it is to mutually support and encourage each other as you work through your grief together.

Ignoring Grief Also Brings Results—Negative Results

If we want to successfully adjust to our hearing loss, we must work through our grief. On the other hand, if we ignore or suppress our grief, it eats away at us on the inside and results in even more serious problems in the future.

We may fear the pain and embarrassment of crying, talking about our losses, or being angry. We've been told that real men don't cry—that they don't show their emotions. (They just die of heart attacks instead.) The only way we get better is by feeling our pain, expressing our feelings to someone who understands, and sharing our grief.[12]

Those people that have the most trouble coping with grief have poor personal and social networks. They don't relate well to others or can't find someone they feel they can relate to. They have few, if any, close personal friends. When loss occurs, they don't have anyone with whom to share their grief.

People also have more trouble coping with grief if they have the added burden of current medical or psychiatric illnesses. If we have too much stress in our lives or have unresolved previous losses we also will have trouble dealing with our current grief.[13]

Here are some common but destructive reactions to grief.

1. Suppressing our emotions.
2. Deliberately keeping too busy so we avoid mourning or remembering the past.
3. Withdrawing from the various activities we once loved.
4. Withdrawing from our family and friends and becoming recluses.

These reactions short-circuit the grieving process. As a result, our emotions do not heal properly. This affects our bodies. It is actually harmful to our health to hold it all in and appear insensitive to our hearing loss. When we do this we are much more susceptible to illness.[14]

Did you know that researchers have linked the development of cancer to unresolved loss? In one study, researchers unexpectedly found that 44 percent of persons with cancer who were referred for counseling had unresolved grief.[15] That's scary. Imagine, by not working through our grief, we could be setting ourselves up for cancer.

Also, unresolved grief is an important factor in alcohol abuse. In one survey, 25 percent of those admitted to an alcohol treatment center had problems handling grief.[16]

Then, too, suppressing grief sometimes results in deep, dark, long-lasting depression. Ignoring grief is just not worth it!

In working through our grief we don't need protection from painful experiences. Rather, we need boldness to face them. We don't need pain killers. We need strength to conquer it.

The Stages of Grief

When we lose some of our hearing loss as adults, many of us experience the same emotional shock and grief we would if we learned that we had a terminal illness.[17] We advance through the various stages of grief—denial, anger, bargaining, depression and acceptance. These stages of grief permit us to recover in due time. Also, understanding these stages helps reassure us that we are not crazy.

> **Where Am I in the Grieving Process?**
>
> We are not necessarily in only one stage of the grieving process at a time. We can be in denial in one aspect of our hearing loss while being perfectly accepting in another aspect. Likewise, we can be angry over one area affected by our lack of hearing and be depressed by another area. To further complicate matters, we can be all of the above at the same time! The ultimate goal, of course, is to reach the acceptance stage for all aspects of our hearing loss.

Chapter 1: Grieving for Your Hearing Loss

We progress through these steps at our own pace. The time it takes for our emotions to heal varies with each of us. This is not a cut and dried process. We may not experience all of these stages of grief, nor necessarily go through them in the same order. Then again, we may regress and go through certain stages all over again. We may get bogged down in one stage or other. Two common ones would be denial and depression. We need to persevere and progress to the next stage until we fully accept our hearing loss. Only then will we find healing and success.[18]

In the next five chapters we will see how each of these stages affect us as we adjust to our hearing loss.

Chapter 1 Endnotes

1. Wright, 1985. pp. 119-136.
2. Barnes, 1989.
3. What Is Grief? 1986.
4. Friio, 1995.
5. Barnes, 1989.
6. Moving Through Grief And Loss, 1988.
7. Worthington, 1994. p. 297.
8. Wright, 1985. pp. 119-136.
9. What Is Grief? 1986.
10. Hawking, 1975.
11. Friio, 1995.
12. Moving Through Grief And Loss, 1988.
13. Barnes, 1989.
14. Krohn, 1989. pp. 197-209.
15. Barnes, 1989.
16. Barnes, 1989.
17. Alpiner, 1987. pp. 435-437.
18. Alpiner, 1987. pp. 435-437.

Chapter 2

Denial

The news shocks us. We express disbelief. "It can't be!" "They're wrong!" "It's not me they are talking about!" "Someone made a mistake!" "I don't have a hearing loss!"

Denial is our first, and I might add, perfectly natural initial reaction when faced with the shocking news we have a hearing loss. Often, it is too painful for us to accept that we will never again hear better than we do now (and our hearing will likely continue to get worse).

We may be shocked numb. The shock temporarily anaesthetizes us—gives us a brief escape from reality. We show little emotion. Later our emotions may boil over. Then we may exhibit anger, anxiety and other strong emotions. Grief pours over us in waves, waxing and waning.[1] This shock stage—in reality it is a counter-shock—may last anywhere from a few minutes to a few hours to a few days.[2]

Denial is the human shock absorber. It is a natural protective mechanism. By temporarily blocking out a loss that's too painful to face, we give ourselves time to adjust gradually to our new reality.[3]

Thus, denial temporarily softens the emotional impact of our hearing loss. Eventually these feelings pass, and we are able to face the reality of our loss.[4]

When we deny that we have a hearing loss, we may pretend that we hear when we don't. We will assert, "I don't have a hearing problem. I hear what I need to hear." We may admit, "Oh, sure, every once in a while I may have a little trouble understanding something, but it's not serious". We may even tell ourselves, "If my hearing ever gets bad, I'm going to do something about it". We may blame others by accusing, "Don't mumble. Speak up!" While we are in this stage, by denying a hearing problem exists, we create other problems for ourselves. Everyday communication becomes frustrating. We need denial—temporarily—but we must not linger on it.

Eventually, it becomes obvious to us that we really do have a hearing loss and cannot deny it any longer. Our next reaction is to deny its permanence. Now instead of saying, "I do not have a hearing loss", we tell ourselves and others that our hearing loss is just temporary. Soon a doctor will discover a miraculous cure, and we will be able to hear normally again.[5]

As long as we deny we have a hearing loss, or deny its permanence, we are not ready to successfully cope with our hearing loss. Of course it's normal to wish the loss never happened. Eventually, when we accept our hearing loss and its permanence, we will be ready and willing to learn how to cope.[6]

At first it is easy to deny we have a hearing loss because often it quietly sneaks up on us. In fact, people who have a mild hearing loss that came on gradually frequently have trouble accepting that they

Chapter 2: Denial

actually have a hearing loss. Because their hearing loss crept up on them imperceptibly over a number of years, they often attribute their trouble hearing to changes in their environment, changes in people, or changes in society in general.

The denial stage can be, and often is, carried to extremes. For example, a wife may point out to her husband that he missed most of the conversation at the meeting they just left. "Nonsense," he replies, "I just didn't want to listen to that old windbag anyway". This type of attitude eventually leads to friction between husband and wife.[7]

Men, more often than women, deny they have a hearing loss. Men often have a difficult time with this stage in the grieving process. Why? Because in our culture, we have been taught that men do not cry. Men do not display weakness. They do not need affection or gentleness. Men do the comforting—they don't need comforting themselves. They help those in need, but do not need help themselves. Men are made out of iron, not flesh. Thus they deny their hearing loss and suffer the consequences.[8]

Some men even go so far as to accuse their wives of having a hearing problem, not them.

Denial of hearing loss is rampant. According to the results of a National Health survey in the US, about 58 percent of people over 65 reported some hearing loss, yet only 8 percent used hearing aids.[9]

Another reason people deny they have a hearing loss is because of the social attitudes shown by hearing people. To them we deviate from normal. We are sub-normal. Consequently, society attaches a stigma to those of us with a hearing loss.

25

> **"Harry"**
>
> "Harry" was concerned that his wife, "Betty," was losing her hearing although Betty heatedly denied it. Exasperated, Harry went to an ear specialist. "Doctor," he said, "What can I do to prove to my wife that she needs to get her hearing attended to?"
>
> The specialist suggested, "Stand some distance behind her and ask her a question. If she doesn't answer, keep moving closer and repeating the question until she answers. Then you will know just how bad her hearing is."
>
> Later, at home, Harry saw Betty making supper at the kitchen counter. From the living room he called, "Honey, what are we having for dinner?" No reply.
>
> He moved to the dining room and called again, "Honey, what are we having for dinner?" Still no reply.
>
> He moved to the kitchen doorway and asked for the third time, "Honey, what are we having for dinner?" He was shocked when again she didn't reply. He had no idea her hearing was **that** bad. So he moved right up behind her and asked once more, "Honey, what are we having for dinner?"
>
> Turning to face him she answered, "Spaghetti and meat balls I said—for the **fourth** time!"

People with normal hearing typically expect those they meet daily will be "normal". They expect the people they meet to speak intelligently and to be able to follow the train of a normal conversation with relative ease. Therefore, they take it for granted that if they speak to us, we will make appropriate replies. They assume that we will take evasive action when they beep their car horns. And they expect that we will respond to our telephones or doorbells. If we deviate from these expectations, they see this handicap as a discreditable stigma.[10]

Historically, physically disabled people have been treated as inferior by "normal" people. Simply put, hearing people have assumed that deaf and hard of hearing people are not fully competent human beings.[11] They equate disability with inability. This is just not true!

For example, Bob, an appliance repair man, answered a call to repair a refrigerator. When his customer noticed he was wearing a hearing aid she immediately became agitated and questioned his qualifications. Why? Because she thought he was incompetent. After all, he was hard of hearing. As he relates, "She believed that because she had a Master's degree she would know more about repairing appliances than a hard of hearing trades person".[12]

As hard of hearing people, we become aware of this stigma when an employer turns us down for a job or promotion. We sense it when people with normal hearing adopt a superior role or display pity or impatience with us. This stigma is emphasized when hearing people label us as "deaf," no matter how poor our hearing is. Many hearing people also believe that deafness is related to daftness. Too often we are stereotyped as slow-thinking and lacking in intelligence. For example, a large study recently revealed that both the intelligence and the personality of hard of hearing people are **always rated less** than that of their hearing peers. It revealed that people associate hearing loss with incompetence, aging, feebleness, impotence, weakness and dumbness.[13]

Many in society still consider us to be both "deaf and dumb," with dumb not meaning mute, but stupid.

Not being able to hear (or speak clearly) is a disability, not senselessness. Yet we are often still treated as if we are "deaf and dumb".[14] For example, one hard of hearing professional recalled, "Once, when I was a social work intern, a patient of mine wondered if I might be mentally retarded (because of her less than perfect speech), but finally decided it was unlikely a mentally retarded person would be working as a psychotherapist!"

Then, too, a hearing loss is not a disability that instinctively appeals to human sympathy. When a person rolls up in a wheelchair, our empathy goes out to him because we realize he is physically disabled. Another person walks in with sunglasses, feeling her way around with a cane. We understand immediately that she is blind and our empathy goes out to her. But then, in walks a person with a hearing loss—looking normal in every other aspect—and we think he is "stupid" because he can't understand us.[15] It is significant that while blind people appear in tragedies, deaf and hard of hearing people are usually made fun of and found in comedies![16]

For example, a hard of hearing joke may be cute, but it probably does not cast us in a particularly good light.

Because the rewards of being considered normal are so great and because the "deaf and dumb" stigma is still so rampant in our society today, many hard of hearing people are strongly tempted to pass themselves off as normally-hearing people! Since, unlike the blind or physically disabled, we have no external symptoms, we can easily hide this fact.

This desire to pass as normal (which we truly are) also explains why many hard of hearing

> **What?**
>
> "Andy" and his wife had fourteen children. One day Joe, his co-worker, asked him why he had so many children.
>
> Replied Andy, "It's because my wife is hard of hearing."
>
> "But what does that have to do with it?" Joe persisted.
>
> "Well," Andy drawled, "Every night when we go to bed I ask my wife, 'Shall we go to sleep or what?' And every night she replies, 'What?'"

people don't wear hearing aids. They regard them as symbols advertising their disability. The alternative is bluffing—pretending we hear when we don't. Bluffing is often our desperate attempt to be accepted as normal, not some abnormal dummy. When bluffing isn't possible, or the strain of pretending becomes too great, we tend to withdraw from society.

It is obvious there are very real reasons for denying we have a hearing loss. Nevertheless, denying we have a hearing loss is a poor response. If we do not express our grief, we may deny that we have been hurt. In a real sense, we are refusing to mourn our loss. If we carry this unfinished business with us, we will suffer unrest, conflict, and ongoing depression. By refusing to mourn, we are refusing to say good-bye to the good hearing we once had.[17] And that makes us angry.

Chapter 2 Endnotes

1. Barnes, 1989.
2. Krohn, 1989. pp. 197-209.
3. Duffy, 1993. p. 86.
4. What Is Grief? 1986.
5. Hardy, 1974. p. 174.
6. Hardy, 1974. p. 175.
7. Rezen, 1985. p. 31.
8. Krohn, 1989. pp. 197-209.
9. Vernick, 1993. p. 39.
10. Higgins, 1980. p. 124.
11. Higgins, 1980. p. 23.
12. Sochowski, 1995. pp. 15-16.
13. Kochkin, 1991. p. 45.
14. Higgins, 1980. p. 135.
15. Chartrand, 1988, p. 7.
16. Lysons, 1978. p. 83.
17. Wright, 1985. pp. 119-136.

Chapter 3

Anger

"Why me?" "It just isn't fair!" "What did I do that I am being punished by having a hearing loss?" "Why did God allow this?" Once we admit we have a hearing loss, we often express rage or anger. This is the second step in the grieving process.

We often question the fairness of having to put up with a hearing loss. We want fairness in life when, in fact, life is unfair (at least from our standpoint). Rather than dwelling on asking why, we need to ultimately accept our situation. Unduly pondering the why leads to destructive behavior. This is a very different process from accepting and grieving our loss. Grief eventually ends. It is a natural process. Wondering why may never end. It is generally unproductive and can lead to bitterness, unhappiness and unnecessary pain. At some point, we must let go of the why, accept the reality, and get on with living.[1]

We may feel robbed, resentful and angry with ourselves or the person or thing that cost us our hearing. We may get stuck here for a time. If we are angry about our hearing loss, we are not yet ready to do anything constructive about it. We need to deal with our anger first. It will take time, but we can work through it.[2]

In our anger we may become aggressive. For example, in the past when I had difficulty following a lecture because the instructor didn't talk loud enough or wore a beard, so I had great difficulty speechreading him, I spent a lot of the time thinking about how poor a teacher he was. I'd think, "The guy must be an idiot if he thinks that he is effectively communicating with his students". This attitude is wrong and doesn't help the situation.

Our anger may be a generalized anger or we may direct it towards a specific person. Most often we vent our aggression on those close to us—like our spouses. This continued anger will strain even the strongest relationship.[3]

How often have we become suspicious and felt people were talking about us when we can't hear the conversation? We may withdraw from conversing with others because we are mad at ourselves when we can't understand speech or mad at them for not speaking up.[4]

Closely associated with anger is guilt. It's not unusual to blame ourselves for something we did or didn't do that may have caused our hearing loss. Sometimes we blame others. Often we blame God. Also, we may feel guilty about some of our other feelings. We spend our time thinking, "If only I had . . ." We need to remember that we are human, and there are events we just can't control.[5]

Because we are angry over losing our hearing we may withdraw from others. When we withdraw from society, we reduce the tension we experience in trying to communicate with others. Then, because we have little interaction with others, we become more and more self-centered. We only think of ourselves and how society is failing us. Instead, we should be going out and working to change society for the better.[6]

In our anger, we may become stubborn, rebellious, abusive and destructive. We may deny the negative traits in ourselves and instead, project them upon others. For example, if we feel inadequate or inferior because of our hearing loss, we project these attitudes upon society as a whole. We say, "It is them, not us, who are really inadequate and inferior."[7]

Chapter 3 Endnotes

1   Friio, 1995.
2   What Is Grief? 1986.
3   Rezen, 1985. p. 32.
4   Alpiner, 1987. pp. 435-437.
5   What Is Grief? 1986.
6   Hardy, 1974. p. 175.
7   Hardy, 1974. pp. 178-179.

Chapter 4

Bargaining

After we quit denying our hearing loss and after our anger has subsided, we may try to bargain our way out of our hearing loss. We are more inclined to bargain if we do not perceive that our hearing loss is permanent. Instead of doing something constructive about our loss, we try to bargain with ourselves or with others. Often we try to strike a deal with God. We say to God, "If you will take this hearing loss away, I will serve you." God rarely responds to this kind of bargain because we should have been doing this in the first place![1,2]

Chapter 4 Endnotes

1   Alpiner, 1987. pp. 435-437.
2   Duffy, 1993. p. 86.

Chapter 5

Depression

Denial has not worked. Anger has not worked. Bargaining has not worked. Thus we conclude that nothing works. Therefore, depression sets in when we finally realize that our hearing loss is real and cannot be reversed. This stage represents a kind of giving up the fight. We acknowledge it is futile. However, this is necessary before we will accept the reality of our loss.[1]

At times our grief may seem like an overwhelming wave, and its strong undercurrents of feelings may make us think we're falling apart. We may be tempted to suppress the pain of grief or mask it with alcohol or drugs. Don't do it. Instead, we need to pour out our sorrow. We need to express our feelings. Don't hold them in. Letting ourselves fully experience our grief is the most effective, healthy way to work through our depression.[2]

Note that we should express our grief to someone with understanding and insight—someone who understands the grieving process. Finding such a person is rare indeed! Could this be why there is so much unresolved grief? The last thing we need to hear from someone who doesn't have a clue what we are going through is, "Buck up. Crying about it isn't going to help matters. You need to pull yourself together." At this moment in our lives we need understanding and sympathy.

We may feel varying degrees of sadness, loneliness and despair. For a time, we may feel physically and mentally drained. We may be unable and unwilling to perform even routine tasks. No, we are not lazy. We are in the middle of grief. That is sapping our energy. We may be restless. We may feel apathy and listlessness—that life is not worth living any more. We may wish we were dead. We may say to ourselves, "I couldn't care less". Thus, our usual activities lose their importance.

We may think about the past and contrast it to a bleak future without our hearing. How will we be able to cope without the full use of one of our two primary senses (sight is the other)? How will we be able to converse in the dark? How will we ever hear on the telephone?[3] Will we ever be able to enjoy music again? Will we be able to delight in jovial company? We know life will be more confusing, difficult and tiring. Just thinking about all this makes us feel sad and depressed.[4]

Our hearing loss may make us feel terribly insecure and isolated. As a result, we may withdraw from social situations that we see as threatening. For example, we may remain aloof so that the others at our table will ignore us. We may pretend to be in a terrible hurry so we have a good excuse not to talk to anyone.[5] This results in a change in our personalities. Our personality changes may leave friends and family frightened of the new person we have become. This may make us feel even more isolated and alone.

Our feelings of depression may be heightened by tinnitus or by undue fatigue caused by the extra energy expended in trying to cope with the demands of an environment in which good hearing is taken for granted.[6]

In our depressed state we may procrastinate and put off doing what we know we should be doing. We may say we are too old to learn how to wear a hearing aid. We may refuse to take a speechreading and coping skills course to help ourselves. We may decide to wait until our hearing loss gets worse before seeking help. We may decide to wait until a better hearing aid comes on the market or the price of hearing aids drops.

We can make any number of excuses why we won't do anything to help our hearing loss. This just results in further depression. We need to realize that unless we take action our hearing loss is going to continue to cause us real problems.

A very real reason for our depression, and one seldom considered by those with normal hearing, is the "dead feeling" that comes from not hearing the background noise that people with normal hearing take for granted. For example, we can be depressed and feel isolated because we no longer hear the everyday sounds of comfort—birds no longer chirp, downtown no longer hums, the wind no longer whistles through the trees, papers do not rustle, people move about silently and dishes and cutlery no longer clink. We feel isolated and out of touch with the world around us. This is depressing to us.[7] We may think, "Everything seems dead, I might as well be dead, too."

We may also feel depressed and insecure because our poor hearing no longer warns us of impending threats such as someone approaching us from behind or someone tampering with the back door. Life becomes full of uncertainty. For example, if we live alone or when we stay in a hotel should we lock the doors? If so, how will someone reach us in an emergency? When we are visiting, we question, "Is the bathroom free?" "Has everyone had breakfast or gone out?" "Is everyone still in bed?" On the highway we wonder how we will manage if we have a breakdown? In group conversations we ask ourselves, "Should I join in or has my remark already been made?" "Is someone still talking?" "Have they changed the subject?"[8]

If we have had good hearing and lost it later in life, we are thoroughly rooted in a hearing society and yet are just as thoroughly blocked from participating in it. Another way of expressing it is, "I am least alone when I am by myself. I am most alone when I am surrounded by people at a dinner or party who leave me out."[9] This is most depressing.

Depression is undesirable and may last for years. Eventually, we take steps—perhaps tiny ones at first—toward becoming involved in life again. As we meet each new little challenge, we learn to handle our feelings of depression.[10] It is only when we finally see chronic depression for what it is—self-imposed exile from the human race—that we can conquer it.

Chapter 5 Endnotes

1   Duffy, 1993. p. 86.
2   Moving Through Grief And Loss, 1988.

Chapter 5: Depression

3 Morton, p. 31.
4 Alpiner, 1987. pp. 435-437.
5 Lysons, 1978. p. 81.
6 Lysons, 1978. pp. 80-81.
7 Rezen, 1985. p. 32.
8 Morton, p. 31.
9 Sherren, p. 38.
10 What Is Grief? 1986.

Chapter 6

Acceptance

The final step is acceptance. At this stage in the grieving process we accept the fact that we have a hearing loss and that our loss is permanent. As we accept this fact, our depression lifts. We begin to say to ourselves, "There is something wrong with my hearing, not with me.[1] I am OK. Only my hearing is impaired, not my intelligence. I may not feel good about being hard of hearing, but I do feel good about myself.[2] I want to live again!"

Now we are ready to take positive steps to deal with our hearing loss. We are no longer willing to miss out on human conversation. We are ready to take charge of our lives and manage our hearing loss. Now we will investigate whether hearing aids will help us hear better. We will enroll in speechreading and hearing loss coping skills classes. We will seek out hearing loss support groups. Now we are ready to be the best hard of hearing people we can be.[3]

This is the only stage where we can effectively deal with the problems of our hearing loss. It may take us from several months and up to two years or more before we reach this stage.

Grieving for Your Hearing Loss

In this stage, the waves of our grief begin to recede and our lives become calmer. The pain becomes less. Gradually hope begins to return. Life will go on. We are now concentrating more on the future than sorrowing over the past.[4] We begin thinking, "I will be able to cope". The changes we have had to make are painful. They take time and are difficult, but they are becoming more natural and habitual. We are growing stronger in the process. We know that we will recover!

We have to adjust to our new level of hearing. We have to struggle with the reality of our new "normal". We have to learn to forgive our own errors and shortcomings. Depending on how we respond to our hearing loss determines whether we come out stronger or weaker.[5]

> **The Choice Is Yours**
>
> Here is how Susan put it, "Life will be as normal as you will let it be—**when you decide** to let it be".

As we begin to adjust to our hearing loss, we may fantasize and in our dream world, put ourselves into many different situations to see how well we will fit in.[6] This is a positive step.

We will begin to look at the positive aspects of our hearing loss. (Surprise! There are some.) For example, we don't have to interrupt a hot bath because now we can't hear the phone ringing. We will also develop in other areas to make up for our lost hearing. It is interesting that several of the speechreading instructors I know were formerly school teachers who can no longer teach in a regular setting because of their hearing loss, but make excellent speechreading and hearing loss coping skills instructors.

Chapter 6: Acceptance

Another step we sometimes take in the path to acceptance of our hearing losses is to identify with a group. In so doing, we reduce our real or perceived inadequacies as we identify with the achievements of the group. This way we offset some of our negative feelings with feelings of worth.[7]

For example, I was a volunteer firefighter in our local Fire/Rescue Company for ten years. I was the only hard of hearing person in this group, but they specifically asked me to join them because of what I could offer them. Although there were certain duties I didn't normally perform because of my lack of hearing, I regularly did most things. Incidentally, in the training courses we took I always graduated near or at the top of the class in spite of my hearing loss.

As we work towards accepting our hearing loss, we often find that the path to our goals is blocked because of our hearing loss. We must not stop there, but try to discover other ways to achieve those or similar goals. Instead of focusing on our shortcomings and defects, we need to focus on our strengths. As we focus on achieving our goals, we will be less concerned with anxieties relating to our hearing loss. This is success.

Unfortunately, no matter how well we cope with our hearing loss, there will be some activities we just won't be able to handle. Our hearing loss doesn't have to hinder our lifestyles. Our lifestyles will change but they need not be any less worthwhile or rewarding.[8]

For example, about 43 years ago I wanted to get my pilot's license and fly. Back then my poor hearing prevented me from passing the pilot's medical. I could have given up right there, but I didn't. I appealed the doctor's decision for two years. Finally, the Department of Transport decided to give me a practical hearing test under real flying conditions. I passed and they amended my medical so that I could obtain a private pilot's license. I became the first person in Canada with a severe hearing loss, as far as the examiners knew, to ever get approval for a private pilot's license! I didn't get all that I wanted—a commercial rating—but I got far more than I would have received otherwise. I could fly!

(Incidentally, today even deaf people can obtain a private pilot's license if they want to. Because they can't hear the radio, they communicate with the control tower with TTY's or follow the rules for landing without radio contact.)

We have finally reached the acceptance stage when we say, "I don't want to miss out on things any more," or "even if I can't hear very well, I still want to enjoy life". Our emotions are now more or less on an even keel. Life is worth living again. Of course we may still have a few bad days from time to time, but we have successfully worked through our grief. We need to congratulate ourselves. We deserve it!

Chapter 6 Endnotes

1. Rezen, 1985. p. 33.
2. Sherren, p. 38.
3. Alpiner, 1987. pp. 435-437.
4. Moving Through Grief And Loss, 1988.
5. Wright, 1985. pp. 119-136.
6. Hardy, 1974. p. 177.
7. Hardy, 1974. p. 179.
8. Rezen, 1985. p. 51.

Chapter 7

Grieving and Your Family

The Rest of Your Family Needs to Grieve Too

Up to now, we have just looked at how hearing loss affects us and our need to grieve for its loss. Unfortunately, however, when hearing loss hits one family member, it affects everyone in the family, not just the person with the hearing loss. Typically, the other family members miss the free and easy (and intimate) conversations they used to have. This saddens and sometimes angers them. Thus, just as for any other kind of loss, they too have to grieve this loss.

Be aware that when parents discover that their child has a hearing loss, it can hit them hard—as it did Tom and his wife—almost as if their child had died. In fact, this is exactly what they may feel—that the "normal" hearing child they gave birth to has "died," leaving in its place a "deaf" child. Thus, their grief is very real, and they need time to grieve.

Hearing loss in the family can hit children hard too. When sudden severe hearing loss hit the mother in one family, her young daughter had a tough time dealing with it. Her daughter remembers the day her mother was taken to the hospital. She sadly lamented,

> "Mommy came back a different mommy. I lost my old mommy. This mommy can't hear. I want my old Mommy back!"

Because she did not have proper support, this little girl regressed. She became a bed wetter and began to have temper tantrums. Thus, when hearing loss hits a family, never forget the needs of the children. They need an external support network to help them through their grief. The reason children need external support is because when their parents are mired in their own grief, they cannot effectively help their children.[1]

If hearing loss hits a spouse, and both do not grieve this loss of communication, it often causes a great strain in the marriage. In fact, unless they work through the grieving process, many marriages do not survive.

Part of the problem is that since both marriage partners need to grieve, they are not available to support each other. The person with the hearing loss is busy grieving and needs support. However, the person they turn too in their grief—their husband or wife—is also grieving, and thus cannot effectively help them. That is why it is **vital** that both the hard of hearing spouse and the hearing spouse **each** have their own support networks to help them successfully navigate the grieving process.

This is what "Sally" and "Bill" did. Sally explained,

Chapter 7: Grieving and Your Family

"Bill and I couldn't support each other in the beginning. We were weighed down by our own sadness and grief. It was like we were sinking because the two of us together were too heavy for our marriage boat. At this point, I turned to my friends, and Bill turned to his. As a result, we stayed together, but we really did have to go outside of our marriage for support."

Where Does Getting Hearing Aids Fit into the Grieving Process?

If your doctor or audiologist has just diagnosed you with a significant hearing loss, **don't** rush out and buy yourself new hearing aids. Pay attention here, because there is a right and a wrong time to get hearing aids. Here's a typical scenario.

You come home with the shocking diagnosis—you have a hearing loss. The first reaction of your hearing family members is to pressure you into getting hearing aids.

Family members, resist this temptation. Yes, your parent/spouse/sibling/child needs hearing aids. However, this is **not** the right time for him/her to get hearing aids. The truth is, millions of dollars of hearing aids lay abandoned in dresser drawers—unwanted and unused—because family members pressured hard of hearing people into getting hearing aids **before** they were ready. Let me explain why in relation to the grieving process.

Denial: Your wife drags you in to have your hearing tested and to hopefully be fitted with hearing aids, because she is convinced you are losing your

Grieving for Your Hearing Loss

hearing. However, as far as you are concerned, it is a total waste of time because you **know** you still hear perfectly fine, so you don't need hearing aids.

Family member, put yourself in the hard of hearing person's shoes. Would you wear hearing aids if you "knew" your hearing was still okay? Of course not! Thus, if you "force" your spouse to get hearing aids, he will often just give his new hearing aids a cursory trial, take them home, toss them in a dresser drawer, and forget all about them. And there goes $5,000.00 down the drain!

Anger: In this stage you are **mad**! When you are mad, you are not thinking rationally. You notice that people aren't speaking up. It's them, not you. You don't need hearing aids! People just need to learn to speak up properly! You think, "Why spend money on hearing aids when my communications problems are not even my fault?"

Bargaining: You have now accepted the fact that you really do have a hearing loss, but you "**know**" this loss is only going to be temporary. You are going to work a deal with the doctors, or maybe even with God Himself, to get your hearing back. Since your hearing loss is going to be temporary, why should you waste good money buying hearing aids you're hardly ever going to use?

Depression: When none of the above works, you become depressed. Since you are depressed, you feel that life is no longer worth living, so what difference does it make whether you hear better or not? Thus, you still won't bother getting or wearing hearing aids.

Chapter 7: Grieving and Your Family

Acceptance: Finally, however, you begin to realize that you **want** to live life to its fullest and in order to do that you want to hear the best you can. It is at this point that you are ready to do whatever it takes in order to hear better. Now is the time for you to hurry to your audiologist for your new hearing aids, because now you are finally ready and willing to give them a fair trial.

Grieving is just the first step on the road to successfully living with your hearing loss. Now that you have successfully worked through your grief, you will be eager to learn more about the rest of the steps that will put you well on your way to successfully living with your hearing loss.

To help you, the author has written the book, "Keys to Successfully Living with Your Hearing Loss". See the back of this book for further information on obtaining this book for yourself.

Chapter 7 Endnotes

1   Bauman, 2011. p. 18-20.

Literature Cited

Alpiner, Jerome G. and Patricia A. McCarthy. 1987. Rehabilitative Audiology: Children And Adults. Williams & Wilkins. Baltimore, MD.

Barnes, Daphne. 1989. The Spectrum Of Grief: Identification And Management. In: *Canadian Family Physician.* Vol. 35. May 1989.

Bauman, Neil. 2011. *Keys to Successfully Living with Your Hearing Loss.* Integrity First Publications. Stewartstown, PA.

Chartrand, Max S. 1988. Psychology Of The Hearing Impaired. Unimax Educational Publications. Texas.

Duffy, Yvonne. 1993. Working Through Grief. In: *Independent Living.* Vol. 8. June, 1993.

Friio, Sam. 1995. Hearing Loss And Grief. Lecture presented to CHIP Instructors. Calgary, Alberta. January, 1995.

Hardy, Richard E. & John G. Cull. 1974. Educational And Psychosocial Aspects Of Deafness. Charles C Thomas, Publisher. Springfield, Illinois.

Hawking, Stephen. 1975. Caltech News. December, 1975.

Higgins, Paul C. 1980. Outsiders In A Hearing World: A Sociology Of Deafness. Sage Publications, Inc. Beverly Hills, California.

Kochkin, Sergei. 1991. What This Industry Needs Is A Marlboro Man. In: *ASHA* (American Speech-Language Hearing Association). December 1991.

Krohn, John. 1989. Crisis Counseling—Death And Grief.

Lysons, Kenneth. 1978. Your Hearing Loss And How To Cope With It. A RNID Handbook. Taken from an abridged version called "Dull Ears." In: *Background Information For Speechreading Instructors*.

Morton, Phyllis. Some Aspects Of Deafness. In: *C.H.I.P. Background Information For Speech Reading Instructors*. Extracted from various issues of the British publication, *Catchword*.

Moving Through Grief And Loss—Understanding The Many Losses We All Face. 1988. Krames Communications. San Bruno, CA.

Rezen, Susan & Carl Hausman. 1985. Coping With Hearing Loss: A Guide For Adults And Their Families. Dembner Books, New York, N.Y.

Sherren, Patricia. Some Thoughts on Being Deaf. In: *C.H.I.P. Background Information For Speech Reading Instructors*. Extracted from various issues of the British publication, *Catchword*.

Sochowski, Robert. 1995. Winds Are Calm. In: *Listen*. Fall, 1995. The Canadian Hard Of Hearing Association. Ottawa, Ontario.

Literature Cited

Vernick, David M. & Constance Grzelka. 1993. The Hearing Loss Handbook. Consumer Reports Books. Yonkers, N.Y.

What Is Grief? 1986. Channing L. Bete Co. Inc. South Deerfield, MA.

Worthington, Ralph C. 1994. Models Of Linear And Cyclical Grief: Different Approaches To Different Experiences. In: *Clinical Pediatrics*, Vol. 33, May 1994.

Wright, H. Norman. 1985. Crisis Counseling—Helping People In Crisis And Stress.

Good Books on Hearing Loss

Integrity First Books in the series:

Everything You Wanted to Know About Your Hearing Loss But Were Afraid to Ask (Because You Knew You Wouldn't Hear the Answers Anyway!)
             by Neil G. Bauman, Ph.D.

If you have enjoyed this book and would like to learn more about hearing loss and how you can successfully live with it, you may be interested in some helpful books by Dr. Neil. Each book is packed with the things you need to know in order to thrive in spite of your various hearing loss issues. The direct link to the following books is at http://hearinglosshelp.com/shop/category/books/.

Ototoxic Drugs Exposed—The Shocking Truth About Prescription Drugs, Medications, Chemicals and Herbals That Can (and Do) Damage Our Ears ($52.45; eBook $39.95)

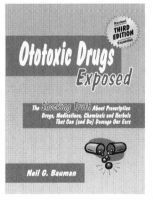

This book, now in its third edition, reveals the shocking truth that many prescription drugs can damage your ears. Some drugs slowly and insidiously rob you of your hearing, cause your ears to ring or destroy your balance. Other drugs can smash your ears in one fell swoop, leaving you with profound, permanent hearing loss and bringing traumatic change into your life. Learn how to protect your ears from the ravages of ototoxic drugs and chemicals. Describes the specific ototoxic effects of 877 drugs, 35 herbals and 148 chemicals (798 pages).

Grieving for Your Hearing Loss

Take Control of Your Tinnitus—Here's How ($29.95; eBook $22.99)

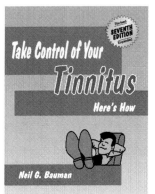

If your ears ring, buzz, chirp, hiss, click or roar, you know just how annoying tinnitus can be. The good news is that you do not have to put up with this racket for the rest of your life. You can take control of your tinnitus. Recent studies show that a lot of what we thought we knew about tinnitus is not true at all. Exciting new research reveals a number of things that you can do to eliminate or greatly reduce the severity of your tinnitus so that it no longer bothers you. This totally-revised, up-to-date and expanded 7th edition contains the very latest in tinnitus research and treatment. In this book you will learn what tinnitus is, what causes tinnitus and things you can do to take control of your tinnitus (356 pages).

Phantom Voices, Ethereal Music & Other Spooky Sounds ($22.49; eBook $16.99)

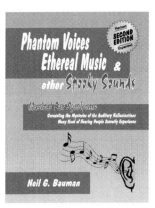

When you realize you are hearing phantom sounds, you immediately think that something has gone dreadfully wrong "upstairs"—that you are going crazy. Because of this, few people openly talk about the strange phantom voices, music, singing and other spooky sounds they hear. This book, the first of its kind in the world, lifts the veil on "Musical Ear syndrome" and reveals numerous first-hand accounts of the many strange phantom sounds people experience. Not only that, it explains what causes these phantom sounds, and more importantly, what you can do to eliminate them, or at least, bring them under control (178 pages).

Say Good Bye to Ménière's Disease—Here's How to Make Your World Stop Spinning ($21.95; eBook $16.49)

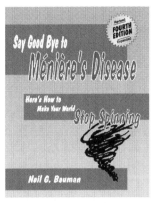

Ménière's disease is one of the more baffling and incapacitating conditions a person can experience. If you suffer from your world spinning, have a fluctuating hearing loss, tinnitus and a feeling of fullness in your ears, this book is for you. It details what Ménière's disease is like; explains the recent breakthrough into the underlying cause of Ménière's; and shows you how, at last, you can be free from the ravages of this debilitating condition. Each page is packed with practical information to help you successfully conquer your Meniere's disease. Join the hundreds and hundreds of people whose worlds have now stopped spinning (128 pages).

Keys to Successfully Living with Your Hearing Loss ($19.97; eBook $15.49)

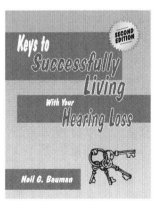

Do you know: a) the critical missing element to successfully living with your hearing loss? b) that the No. 1 coping strategy hard of hearing people instinctively use is wrong, wrong, wrong? c) what the single most effective hearing loss coping strategy is? d) how you can turn your hearing aids into awesome hearing devices? This book addresses the surprising answers to these and other critical questions. Applying them to your life will put you well on the road to successfully living with your hearing loss. (84 pages).

Help! I'm Losing My Hearing—What Do I Do Now? ($18.95; eBook $14.49)

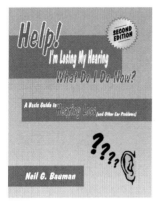

Losing your hearing can flip your world upside down and leave your mind in a turmoil. You may be full of fears, wondering how you will be able to live the rest of your life as a hard of hearing person. You don't know where to turn. You lament, "What do I do now?" Set your mind at rest. This easy to read book, written by a fellow hard of hearing person, is packed with the information and resources you need to successfully deal with your hearing loss and other ear conditions. (116 pages).

Grieving for Your Hearing Loss—The Rocky Road from Denial to Acceptance ($12.95; eBook $9.95)

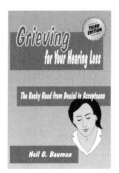

When you lose your hearing you need to grieve. This is not optional—but critical to your continued mental and physical health. This book leads you through the process of dealing with the grief and pain you experience as a result of your hearing loss. It explains what you are going through each step of the way. It gives you hope when you are in the depths of despair and depression. It shows you how you can lead a happy vibrant life again in spite of your hearing loss. This book has helped many (56 pages).

Good Books on Hearing Loss

Talking with Hard of Hearing People—Here's How to Do It Right! ($9.95; eBook $7.95)

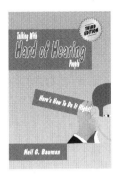

Talking is important to all of us. When communication breaks down, we all suffer. For hard of hearing people this happens all the time. This book is for you—whether you are hearing or hard of hearing! It explains how to communicate with hard of hearing people in one-to-one situations, in groups and meetings, in emergency situations, and in hospitals and nursing homes. When you use the principles given in this book, good things will happen and you will finally be able to have a comfortable chat with a hard of hearing person (38 pages).

When Hearing Loss Ambushes Your Ears—Here's What Happens When Your Hearing Goes on the Fritz ($14.95; eBook $11.95)

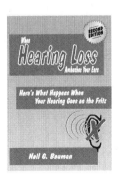

Hearing loss often blind-sides you. As a result, your first step should be to learn as much as you can about your hearing loss; then you will be able to cope better. This most interesting book explains how your ears work, the causes of hearing loss, what you can expect to hear with different levels of hearing loss and why you often can't understand what you hear. Lots of audiograms and charts help make things clear. You will also discover a lot of fascinating things about how loud noises damage your ears (88 pages).

Supersensitive to Sound? You May Have Hyperacusis ($9.95; eBook $7.95)

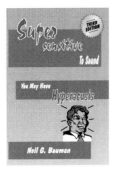

If some (or all) normal sounds seem so loud they blow your socks off, this is the book you want to read! You don't have to avoid noise or lock yourself away in a soundproof room. Exciting new research on this previously baffling problem reveals what you can do to help bring your hyperacusis under control (42 pages).

Here! Here! You and Your Hearing Loss/You and Your Hearing Aids ($12.95; eBook $10.95)

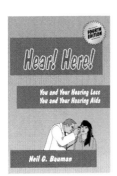

Part I of this book contains a series of my newspaper articles on hearing loss such as, "Hear Today. Gone Tomorrow?" "Hearing Loss Is Sneaky!" "The Wages of Din Is Deaf!" "When Your Ears Ring..." "Get In My Face Before You Speak!" "How's That Again?" "Being Hard of Hearing Is Hard" "I'm Deaf, Not Daft!" Part II contains articles on hearing aids such as, "You Better Watch Out..." "Before Buying Your First Hearing Aid..." "Please Don't Lock Me Away in Your Drawer" "Good-bye World of Silence!" "Becoming Friends with Your Hearing Aids" "Two's Better Than One!" (56 pages).

You can order any of the foregoing books/eBooks (plus you can read more than 1,000 other helpful articles about hearing loss and related issues) from the
Center for Hearing Loss Help
web site at
http://hearinglosshelp.com
or order them from the address below

Center for
Hearing Loss Help

1013 Ridgeway Drive,
Lynden, WA 98264-1057
Phone: (360) 778-1266
FAX: (360) 389-5226
E-mail: info@hearinglosshelp.com
Web site: http://hearinglosshelp.com

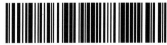

Made in the USA
Columbia, SC
23 September 2018